The Owner's Living Chip Manual

A Humorous, Practical Guide to Upgrading Your Health

Steven Warren, MD, DPA

and

Darren Lopez, MBA

Regenerative Wellness Center

HappyMD.co

The Owner's Living Chip Manual

A Humorous, Practical Guide to Upgrading Your Health

Published by Regenerative Wellness Center

HappyMD.co

ISBN (Paperback): 978-1-972800-08-9

ISBN (Ebook): 978-1-972800-09-6

Disclaimer: This booklet is for educational purposes only and does not constitute medical advice. Always consult a qualified healthcare provider before starting any new health program, supplement regimen, or medication.

First Edition, 2026

Printed in the United States of America

Table of Contents

Imagine you just opened a new phone and found a note inside that says, "This device can last 100 years if used as directed."

Welcome to your Living Chip: the built-in operating system that runs your body, mind, and energy every day.

No one gave you a real owner's manual at birth. Instead, you picked up random "installation files" from parents, friends, TikTok, and the snack aisle. Some of those files were useful; some were... viruses in fancy packaging.

Your Living Chip is always listening. Every bite you eat, every night you sleep—or don't—every walk, worry, and workout is a software update. Tiny choices send tiny signals that say, "Please repair," "Please inflame," or "Please store this as belly fat for the next famine that never comes."

The good news is: your chip is incredibly forgiving. You can ship a new version any time. You don't need to be perfect; you just need to start sending better instructions, more often than not.

In this booklet, you'll learn how to:

- Understand your basic "hardware" (your body).
- Update your "software" (your habits and mindset).
- Write a simple "user manual" for Future You.

Think of this as a friendly, no-judgment manual that says, "Here's how to keep this amazing device—yourself—running smoother, longer, and with more joy."

Chapter 2 — Meet Your User: Present You and Future You

Every device has a user. In this story, the user is... you. Actually, there are two versions of you: Present You and Future You.

Present You is the one who wants chips now, Netflix now, and bed "later." Future You is the one who has to wear Present You's choices. Present You says, "One more episode." Future You says, "Why do I feel like warmed-over roadkill at 6 a.m.?"

Here's the twist: they are both you, and they are both trying to help. Present You wants comfort and relief; Future You wants freedom and health. Life feels better when they work as a team instead of enemies.

Try this simple mental trick:

- Before a choice, pause for two seconds.
- Imagine Future You 24 hours from now.
- Ask, "What tiny upgrade would make their day easier?"

It might be one glass of water. It might be walking five minutes after dinner. It might be turning off your screen 15 minutes earlier.

These are not life-overhauls; they're micro-gifts you send forward in time. The Living Chip loves small consistent upgrades more than heroic, short-lived efforts. Think "version 1.1," not "I must become a completely different person by Monday."

Chapter 3 — Upgrade Your Hardware: Body Basics

Your body is the hardware your Living Chip runs on. If the hardware is inflamed, exhausted, or under-fueled, even the best "apps" crash. Four big levers make the biggest difference: sleep, movement, food, and stress.

Sleep: Night-Shift Repair Crew

At night, a tiny repair crew clocks in. They clean up brain waste, balance hormones, and file memories. When you cut sleep, you cut maintenance.

Aim for a steady sleep window most nights, like 10:30 p.m. to 6:00 a.m. Keep the room cool, dark, and boring. If your phone is the last face you see at night, it will not write you a good performance review in the morning.

Tiny upgrades you can start this week:

- Move screens 15–30 minutes earlier.
- Dim lights an hour before bed.
- Have a simple wind-down ritual: stretch, read, breathe.

Movement: Keep the Pump Running

You are not a parked car; you are closer to a circulating fountain. Blood, lymph, and nutrients move better when you do. The human body was not designed for 10 hours of chair time.

You don't need intense workouts to send a "we are alive and thriving" signal. Standing up every 30–60 minutes, walking after meals, and using stairs are all valid updates.

Tiny upgrades:

- Add a 5–10 minute walk after one meal per day.
- Stand or walk during one phone call.
- Think "move more often," not "exercise or fail."

Food: Fuel, Not Punishment

Your chip reads food as information. Ultra-processed food screams, "Store fat, inflame, feel foggy." Whole, colorful food whispers, "Repair, energize, stabilize."

You don't need a perfect diet; you need a better default.

Tiny upgrades:

- Add one serving of plants to a meal you already eat.
- Swap one sugary drink for water, tea, or sparkling water.
- Keep tempting snacks off your desk and out of arm's reach.

Stress: Your Alarm System

Stress is your built-in alarm system. It's useful when a car is coming at you, less useful when an email is. If the alarm never shuts off, the system wears down.

You may not control all stress, but you can control how long it lives in your body.

Tiny upgrades:

- Take three slow breaths before you answer a stressful message.
- Have a 30-second "reset ritual" (stand up, stretch, look out a window).
- Write worries down instead of letting them spin in your head.

At the end of this chapter, pick one micro-upgrade in each category, not ten. The Living Chip responds beautifully to "small, steady, and kind."

Chapter 4 — Upgrade Your Software: Habits and Mindset

If hardware is your body, software is your habits and stories. Many of us are running "Version 0.9: Makes Life Harder Than Necessary." The goal is not perfection; it's smoother defaults.

Tiny Habits Beat Giant Intentions

"I'll run five miles every day at 5 a.m. starting tomorrow" is a lovely fantasy and a terrible software update. Your brain reads that as "Threat detected."

Instead, shrink the habit until it feels almost silly:

- "I will put on my walking shoes and go to the mailbox."
- "I will fill a glass of water when I start the coffee maker."
- "I will stretch for one minute before bed."

You can always do more once you start, but you win as soon as you do the tiny version. Habits grow from consistent wins, not occasional heroics.

Identity: Who You Believe You Are

Behavior sticks better when it matches identity. "I'm trying to be healthy" is fragile. "I'm the kind of person who walks after dinner" is stronger.

Choose one simple identity sentence today:

- "I am the kind of person who takes care of Future Me."
- "I am the kind of person who moves my body every day."
- "I am the kind of person who goes to bed on purpose, not by accident."

Read it out loud once a day. Then look for tiny actions that prove it true.

When You Fall Off the Habit Ladder

You will miss days. You will eat the thing, skip the walk, or doom-scroll until midnight. That does not mean the update failed; it means you are human.

The only rule that matters here is: never miss twice on purpose. If today went off the rails, tomorrow is not ruined. You just climb back onto the lowest step: the tiny version.

Your Living Chip does not keep a moral scorecard. It keeps a running average.

Chapter 5 — Writing Your Owner's Manual

Now it's time to turn ideas into your personal "Owner's Manual." This is not a legal document; it's a friendly agreement between Present You and Future You.

You can keep it on one page. Write in pen, pencil, or crayon if you like. The important thing is that it is yours.

Use these prompts:

1. **"When I feel my best, my day usually includes..."**
    - Example: "A decent night of sleep, at least one walk, something green on my plate, and one quiet moment."
2. **"My default settings I want to change are..."**
    - Example: "Staying up 'just one more episode,' snacking when I'm stressed, sitting all afternoon without moving."
3. **"My tiny upgrades for the next 7 days are..."**
    - One sleep upgrade: "Screens off 15 minutes earlier."
    - One movement upgrade: "Walk 5 minutes after lunch."
    - One food upgrade: "Add one fruit or vegetable to breakfast."
    - One stress upgrade: "Three slow breaths before I open my email."

4. **"My identity statement is..."**
    - "I am the kind of person who takes small daily steps to protect my future health."

Put this page somewhere you will see it daily. You are not signing up for a boot camp; you are signing up for a kinder relationship with your own Living Chip.

This is version 1.0 of your manual. You will update it as you learn what works. Your body will keep listening, your chip will keep adapting, and Future You will keep whispering, "Thank you."

Chapter 6 — Tools for Your Living Chip: Inside-Out Upgrades

In the earlier chapters, you learned how your daily choices are software updates for your Living Chip. Food, sleep, movement, and stress management will always be the foundation.

Sometimes, though, we want extra tools—targeted products that help the chip run more efficiently or make behavior change easier to sustain. This chapter is about how to plug those tools into the system you already learned, not to replace the basics.

Think of these as "helpers," not heroes. They work best when they ride on top of real-world habits, not instead of them.

The 24-Hour Cell Support System (UCOS and the 365 Line)

Your cells are like tiny factories that never close. They need energy, clean-up crews, and good communication to keep you moving, thinking, and repairing.

The Ultimate Cellular Optimization System (UCOS) from HappyMD.co is designed as a 24-hour support loop for those cellular factories. Different pieces are targeted for different parts of your day and different cellular jobs.

Think of the day in three phases:

- Morning: "Turn the lights on in the factory." Products here focus on energy, mitochondrial support, and getting the system out of 'idle' and into 'ready.'
- Midday: "Keep the line running smoothly." Support for resilience, focus, and metabolic balance while you are active.
- Evening and night: "Repair, restore, and take out the trash." Products aimed at recovery, cellular cleanup, and quality sleep support.

Here's a simple day-in-the-life example:

"At breakfast I take my morning UCOS stack with a glass of water and protein. At lunch I use my midday support with my main meal. In the evening I take my restore products 60–90 minutes before bed as part of my wind-down ritual."

These products help the Living Chip make better use of the lifestyle changes you're already making, especially around energy, recovery, and metabolic health.

NAD+ Support — Powering the Battery (The 2026 Science)

Inside every cell, NAD+ is a critical co-factor that helps turn food into usable energy and supports repair processes. Levels tend to decline with age and metabolic stress, which is why there is so much interest in NAD+-boosting strategies.

Why We Use True-Form NAD+, Not Precursors

If you've shopped for "NAD+ supplements" online, you've probably seen bottles labeled NR (nicotinamide riboside) or NMN (nicotinamide mononucleotide). They're marketed as NAD+ boosters. They are not NAD+. They are precursors—raw materials your body is supposed to convert into NAD+ after you swallow them.

Here's the problem: the science of 2025–2026 has shown us that conversion is far messier than anyone thought.

What Actually Happens When You Swallow NR or NMN

A landmark head-to-head human trial published in Nature Metabolism in January 2026 compared NR, NMN, and nicotinamide (NAM) directly in healthy adults. The findings were striking: NR and NMN are not directly absorbed into the bloodstream as intact molecules. Instead, they are retained in the gut, broken down by your intestinal bacteria, and converted into nicotinic acid (NA)—a much simpler compound—before they ever reach your blood.

In other words, when you swallow an NR or NMN capsule, your gut bacteria have to do the heavy lifting. The precursor you paid for is disassembled in your intestines, converted by microbes into a different molecule, and only then does that molecule boost your NAD+ levels through an indirect pathway.

A comprehensive mouse study published in Science Advances in March 2025 confirmed this further: only a small portion of orally administered NMN and NR was directly absorbed from the small intestine. The vast majority underwent gut microbiota-mediated deamidation and conversion to nicotinic acid. When the researchers used germ-free mice (animals with no gut bacteria at all), the NAD+ increase from oral NR and NMN was significantly suppressed—proving the microbiome is not optional in this process; it is required.

The Microbiome Problem

This creates a serious real-world issue: your results from NR or NMN depend heavily on the health and composition of your gut microbiome.

If your microbiome is disrupted—by antibiotics, ultra-processed food, chronic stress, GLP-1 medications that alter gut motility, or simply aging—your ability to convert those precursors into usable NAD+ may be compromised.

You could be taking an expensive NMN capsule every morning and getting a fraction of the NAD+ you think you're getting, because the bacterial workforce responsible for converting it isn't showing up.

Why We Chose True-Form Sublingual NAD+ (MODS MAX Technology)

In this clinic, we use food-grade, true-form NAD+ delivered sublingually—under the tongue—in our MODS MAX products (Activate365, Mito365, Renew365, NAD+ PQQ Boost).

What MODS MAX Actually Does

MODS MAX stands for Mineral Oxide Delivery System. It is a patented/patent-pending technology from Best 365 Labs that transiently enhances mucosal and GI absorption by opening tight junctions throughout the GI tract. Think of tight junctions like the turnstiles at a stadium. Most oral supplements can't get through them, so they end up going around the long way—and most of the active ingredient never makes it to your bloodstream. MODS MAX briefly opens those turnstiles.

Most oral supplements achieve only 10–15% absorption. MODS MAX dramatically improves uptake—and the sublingual products act as "primers" that activate the absorption window before the tablets arrive.

The Protocol Order Matters

- Sublingual primers first: Activate365 (morning) or Restore365 (evening) are held under the tongue for 30 seconds. They activate the MODS MAX absorption window.
- Tablets follow: Mito365 and Renew365 are taken right after the sublingual primer, riding the enhanced absorption window for significantly improved uptake of

NAD+, CoQ10, PQQ, methylene blue, and the other active ingredients.

This matters for three reasons:

- It bypasses the gut and the liver entirely. The sublingual mucosa is highly vascularized. When NAD+ dissolves under your tongue, it enters the bloodstream directly, skipping stomach acid, intestinal bacteria, and the first-pass liver metabolism that destroys most oral supplements.
- It delivers NAD+ as NAD+—not a precursor that needs conversion. A 2024 pharmacokinetic study on sublingual NAD+ demonstrated for the first time that NAD+ can directly enter cells, most probably via connexin 43 hemichannels and solute carrier channels. Plasma NAD+ levels doubled within 10 minutes of sublingual dosing, with approximately 22% bioavailability compared to IV administration.
- It removes the microbiome variable. Because sublingual delivery skips the gut entirely, it doesn't matter whether your microbiome is in perfect shape or disrupted. You get consistent, predictable NAD+ delivery every single day.

Daily Matters More Than Occasional

NAD+ is consumed constantly by your cells—by sirtuins regulating gene expression, by PARP enzymes repairing DNA, by CD38 in immune signaling. It is not a nutrient you can "load up" once a week and coast.

Your Living Chip needs a steady, daily signal. That's why our protocol is built around daily sublingual dosing, not occasional mega-doses or IV-only approaches:

- Activate365 delivers 20 mg NAD+ every morning as your baseline "oil change."
- Mito365 adds 150 mg NAD+ with PQQ, methylene blue, copper peptide, and B12 for a robust mitochondrial push.
- Renew365 provides 200 mg NAD+ with CoQ10 and fisetin for longevity and senolytic support.
- NAD+ PQQ Boost delivers 200 mg NAD+ with PQQ as a pure mitochondrial accelerator.

When stacked in our core protocol (Mito365 150 mg + Renew365 200 mg + Activate365 20 mg), daily NAD+ intake totals 370 mg—delivered directly, consistently, and without depending on your gut bacteria to do the conversion.

IV NAD+ infusions remain an excellent tool for periodic "deep service" sessions, but they are not a replacement for daily sublingual support. Think of IV days as the deep soak and daily sublinguals as the steady rain.

The Bottom Line

The old model said: "Take an NR or NMN capsule, your body will figure it out." The 2025–2026 science says: "Your gut bacteria have to convert those precursors first, and that process is inconsistent, incomplete, and microbiome-dependent."

We've moved past that model. In this clinic, we deliver true-form NAD+ sublingually so it reaches your bloodstream and your cells directly, daily, and reliably—regardless of your gut health, your medications, or your age. That is the 2026 standard. That is what your Living Chip deserves.

GLP-1 / Semaglutide-Type Medications — Rewriting Appetite Signals

For some people, especially those with obesity or high cardiometabolic risk, the Living Chip's appetite and weight-regulation software has been pushed far off center. In these cases, medications like semaglutide can be powerful tools to help reset the system.

Large, long-term trials show that semaglutide can help patients lose around 10% of their body weight over several years and reduce waist circumference by several centimeters. It also improves cardiometabolic risk factors—including blood pressure, fasting glucose, and lipids—and reduces major cardiovascular events in high-risk patients.

In the language of this booklet:

- Semaglutide is a "signal re-writer" for hunger and fullness.
- It can lower the volume on cravings and make it easier to follow the lifestyle plan you already designed.
- The medication works best when you are also updating your hardware and software: food environment, movement, sleep, and stress.

Here's the honest truth about appetite and weight:

"If your appetite software has been overwhelmed by years of modern food and stress, you are not broken. Tools like GLP-1 medications can help lower the background noise so you can actually hear your body's signals again. We pair them with a personalized plan for movement, nutrition, and sleep so the benefits are real and sustainable."

You can also reassure them that benefits are not only about the scale; semaglutide has been shown to reduce cardiovascular events in people with overweight or obesity, even when weight loss is modest.

Putting It All Together — A Simple Daily Map

Morning

- Wake at a consistent time, get light exposure, move 5–10 minutes.

- Start with Activate365 sublingual (1 mL, hold 30 seconds under tongue), then take Mito365 + Renew365 tablets with or without food.
- If on GLP-1 therapy, follow prescribed timing and injection instructions.

Midday

- Walk after one meal if possible.
- Take midday cellular support as directed.
- Use one stress reset: three slow breaths, a brief pause before going back to work.

Evening

- Aim for an eating window that ends 2–3 hours before bed, as medically appropriate.
- Take Restore365 sublingual 30–60 minutes before bed, then follow with TPrime365 sublingual.
- Start your wind-down routine: lower lights, screens off earlier, simple stretching.

Ongoing

- If using NAD+ support, follow timing and dosing set by your clinician and review labs and how you feel at regular intervals.
- If using GLP-1 therapy, monitor appetite, GI symptoms, and metabolic markers with your care team.

Remember: these tools are optional modules. The core message remains: the Living Chip thrives on consistent, compassionate care. Products and medications can be excellent allies, but you—the user—are still the most important part of the system.

Chapter 7 — The Living Chip Toolbox: How All the Products Fit Your Plan

You've met your Living Chip, your hardware, and your habits. Now let's talk about the "toolbox" of products we sometimes use to support your cells, metabolism, hormones, brain, hair, and more.

These tools do not replace real life. They are there to make the healthy life you want easier, more effective, and more sustainable. Think of them as upgrades that help your system respond better to the work you're already doing.

We'll walk through:

- Daily cell and energy support
- Weight-loss / GLP-1 support packs
- Testosterone and hormone support
- Hair restoration tools
- Longevity bundles
- IV therapy as an occasional "deep service"

You and I will choose only what you actually need. No one needs everything.

1. Daily Cell Support — The 365 "Engine Room"

These products are your core "engine and repair" helpers. They support energy, mitochondria, and recovery.

Activate365 — "Daily oil change." Sublingual morning liquid. NAD+ 20 mg for cellular energy, spermidine for cellular cleanup, boron for hormone metabolism. This is the morning primer that activates the MODS MAX absorption window.

Mito365 — "Powerhouse matrix." Morning tablets, usually after Activate365. NAD+ 150 mg, PQQ to help build new mitochondria, methylene blue 10 mg (delivered as 2 x 5 mg), GHK-Cu copper peptide for tissue repair and collagen support, plus B12 for nerve health. This is often the one people notice in their energy and focus.

MitoBoost Ultra — "Energy and stress shield." Morning tablets. Ashwagandha for cortisol support, methylene blue and PQQ for mitochondrial energy. A go-to when someone feels exhausted and stressed.

Metabolism+ — "Thermogenic focus." Morning tablets. Designed to support metabolism, especially when you're on GLP-1 medications or cutting calories: EGCG and guarana for burn, L-theanine to avoid jitters, low-dose methylene blue for clean focus.

Restore365 — "Sleep optimizer." Sublingual liquid 30–60 minutes before bed. GABA 50 mg for calming, physiologic-dose melatonin (not the mega-doses that leave you groggy), boron and zinc for overnight hormone and repair support. The evening MODS MAX primer.

Renew365 — "Senolytic longevity." Daily tablets focused on longer-term healthspan. NAD+ 200 mg, CoQ10 200 mg, pterostilbene 100 mg, and fisetin 40 mg—for senolytic action (zombie cell cleanup), mitochondrial energy, and cardiovascular support.

MB12+LM — "B12 + minerals safety net." Daily liquid, oral or sublingual. High-dose methylated B12, especially important for patients on GLP-1 medications and those at risk for deficiency.

NAD+ PQQ Boost — "Mitochondrial accelerator." Morning tablets. Pure NAD+ + PQQ combo for strong mitochondrial support and insulin sensitivity.

NeuroPro Plus — "Brain and night support." Evening tablet. Lower-dose methylene blue plus vitamin C to support overnight neuronal mitochondria and brain repair.

These pieces are often combined into bundles so you don't have to think about every bottle individually. Next, we'll see how they plug into specific goals.

2. GLP-1 Weight-Loss Packs — Protecting Muscle, Metabolism, and Brain

If you're using a GLP-1 medication like semaglutide for weight loss, the goal is not just "lose pounds." We want to protect muscle, mitochondria, and brain function while fat is coming off.

There are three GLP-1 packs:

GLP-1 Pack 1 — "Muscle & Metabolism Shield" (Flagship). Morning: Activate365, Mito365, Metabolism+. Evening: Restore365. Maintains muscle and metabolic rate while you eat less, protects energy and focus, improves sleep and overnight repair.

GLP-1 Pack 2 — "Energy & Muscle Insurance" (Simple starter). Morning: MitoBoost Ultra + MB12+LM. Supports cortisol and stress, protects nerves and energy (B12), simple 2-product option for new GLP-1 users or budget-sensitive patients.

GLP-1 Pack 3 — "Diet Accelerator + Brain Protection." Morning: NAD+ PQQ Boost + MB12+LM. Evening: NeuroPro Plus. Strong mitochondrial support for fat burning, B12 safety net, night-time brain and mitochondrial repair.

"GLP-1 medications help control appetite and blood sugar. These packs help protect what you want to keep—muscle, mitochondria, and brain—while we're intentionally losing fat."

3. Testosterone / Hormone Packs — Repairing the Hormone "Signal System"

For men with low testosterone or symptoms of hormonal imbalance, there are several paths. We always start with your labs, symptoms, goals, and fertility needs.

Key tools:

NHTO (Non-Hormonal Testosterone Optimizer, Rx) — Sublingual liquid with enclomiphene, boron, and vitamin C. Signals your own testicular production (supports LH/FSH), preserves fertility. Used in men who want to increase T without shutting down sperm production.

Testosterone Cypionate (Rx) — Injectable testosterone, usually every 3.5 days for steady levels. For men who truly need direct hormone replacement and are comfortable with fertility trade-offs.

TRT Packs:

TRT Pack 1 — "Natural + UCOS." NHTO + Activate365 + Mito365 + Restore365. Boosts your own testosterone signal while supporting cellular energy and sleep while hormones normalize.

TRT Pack 2 — "Performance Stack." Testosterone Cypionate + Activate365 + MitoBoost Ultra + Mito365 + Renew365. Full TRT plus heavy mitochondrial and longevity support.

TRT Pack 3 — "Metabolic / Stress / Recovery." NHTO + Metabolism+ + MitoBoost Ultra + MB12+LM. Addresses low T, slowed metabolism, high cortisol, and B12 needs all at once.

"We're not chasing a number; we're restoring a signal. These packs combine hormone support with cellular and metabolic support so you feel better and protect long-term health, not just your lab report."

TPrime365 — Testosterone Signal Booster

Think of your body's testosterone production like a dimmer switch. The power was always there—TPrime365 just turns it up. It doesn't inject external testosterone. It signals your body to produce more of its own.

TPrime365 (Men) — "Testosterone Signal Booster." Sublingual liquid, 1 mL held 30 seconds under the tongue. Evening dosing: taken right after Restore365, 30–60 minutes before bed. Uses MODS MAX absorption technology for direct sublingual uptake. Contains enclomiphene citrate—a non-hormonal testosterone optimizer that works with your body's own LH/FSH signaling pathway. Preserves fertility. Supports energy, mood, bone strength, muscle tone, libido, and mental clarity. Requires a prescription—ask your provider or visit HappyMD.co.

TPrime365 Women — "Hormone Harmony" (Coming Soon). TPrime365 for Women is in development and will be available at HappyMD.co. The female version is specially formulated for women's hormonal needs, supporting energy, mood, bone density, and healthy aging. DHEA supports bone density, immune function, mood, and healthy aging in women. Same MODS MAX sublingual delivery.

You are not a bundle; you are a human with a Living Chip that wants to thrive. This toolbox is here to help that happen with more ease, faster repair, and better long-term health.

Chapter 8 — Your Metabolic Story: Weight, Energy, and Appetite

Your weight is not a moral report card. It is a story about signals: food signals, stress signals, sleep signals, hormone signals, and genetics all talking at once.

When modern life turns the volume up on ultra-processed food, sitting, stress, and poor sleep, your Living Chip does exactly what it was designed to do: it protects you by storing energy for later. The problem is, "later" never comes. So the storage tanks fill, and you feel heavier, slower, and more frustrated than lazy.

In this program we treat weight as information, not accusation. We ask questions like:

- How hungry are you at different times of day?
- What happens to your energy after meals?
- How do you sleep?
- What meds, life events, or hormones might be nudging the chip off center?

We then choose tools to match your story:

- Lifestyle levers: how you eat, move, sleep, and decompress.
- Cellular support: products that protect muscle and mitochondria when you're losing fat.

- Signal re-writers: GLP-1 medications or hormone therapy when the built-in software is deeply out of tune.

Your only job is honesty and curiosity. My job is to help you write a new metabolic story that you can actually live inside.

Chapter 9 — Your GLP-1 Game Plan: Losing Fat, Keeping You

If we decide together that a GLP-1 medication (like semaglutide) is appropriate, we are not just "putting you on a shot." We are building a game plan that protects the parts of you we want to keep while we lose the fat we don't.

GLP-1 medications help by:

- Turning down the constant "food noise."
- Slowing stomach emptying so you feel full on less food.
- Improving blood sugar control and cardiometabolic risk.

Here's how we frame it in this clinic:

We protect muscle and mitochondria. That's why we give you specific support packs, like the GLP-1 Packs that combine mitochondrial support, B12, and metabolic helpers. We also ask you to move your body, especially with some resistance work, so your muscles stay online while fat goes away.

We protect your brain and mood. Appetite changes can be emotionally weird; your old coping patterns may not fit. Certain products support brain energy at night, and we talk openly about mood, stress, and identity as your body changes.

We protect your relationship with food. We are not aiming for a lifetime battle with your plate. While your appetite is quieter, we practice new defaults: more protein and plants, fewer ultra-processed foods, regular mealtimes, and gentle boundaries around eating windows.

"The medication turns down the volume. Your habits and our mitochondrial support turn up your health. Our shared goal is not just a smaller body; it's a more capable life."

Over time, we periodically reassess: Is your weight still changing in a healthy direction? How are your labs? How do you feel in your own skin? Together we decide whether to stay, step down, or step off, always with a plan.

Chapter 10 — Hormones and Vitality: Turning the Lights Back On

Hormones are your body's text messages. When they're clear and timely, you feel like yourself. When they're scrambled or muted, you feel "off" in ways that are hard to explain.

For men with low or borderline-low testosterone, the symptoms can include:

- Low energy and stamina
- Reduced strength or slower recovery
- Low libido or changes in erections
- Brain fog, irritability, or flat mood
- Increased belly fat and lost muscle

In this clinic we have two main approaches:

Wake up your own signal. Using non-hormonal tools like NHTO, we can sometimes get your own testes to make more testosterone again while preserving fertility. We pair that with mitochondrial and sleep support so your cells can actually use the hormone signal you're sending.

Replace the signal directly. When appropriate, we use testosterone cypionate injections to restore levels in men whose systems truly cannot keep up. We talk clearly about trade-offs, including effects on fertility, and we monitor labs, symptoms, and body composition over time.

Either way, the goal is not "high numbers at any cost." The goal is aligned signals: hormones, sleep, movement, nutrition, and stress all pointing in the same direction.

We often combine hormone support with specific packs that protect mitochondria and heart health, support stress resilience and metabolism, and promote better sleep and long-term healthspan.

You are not "cheating" by using these tools. You are giving your Living Chip the signals it was meant to receive, in an environment it was never designed for.

Chapter 11 — Hair, Skin, and Confidence: Your Outside Tells a Story Too

Your Living Chip doesn't stop at your heart and liver. It also runs your hair follicles, skin cells, and nails—tiny billboards of how your internal world is doing.

When hair starts thinning or skin looks dull, it's rarely "just cosmetic." It can be an early whisper about stress, hormones, nutrition, mitochondrial energy, or local blood flow.

We treat hair and skin as part of your whole-system health:

- We make sure your foundation is solid: protein intake, key nutrients, sleep, stress, and hormones.
- Then we add targeted tools that deliver better signals and fuel to the places you see in the mirror.

You're allowed to care about how you look. It's not vanity—it's feedback, and it often drives the motivation to improve the rest of your health too.

The Hair Tools: What We Actually Use

Marc Ward's Design Chemistry lab formulates our topical hair products around one idea: wake up the follicle's own cellular machinery before you try to grow anything.

JXL-069 spray — Daily topical. Non-hormonal metabolic wake-up signal for dormant follicles. Think of it as ringing the doorbell before you try to walk in.

Scalp MODS serum — Topical serum applied after microneedling when skin channels are open. Contains NAD+, PQQ, methylene blue, copper peptide (GHK-Cu), niacinamide, and hyaluronic acid for local mitochondrial support and scalp hydration.

Hair Growth Serum — Features Redensyl (a patented DHQG+EGCG2 compound shown in studies to be 214% more effective than minoxidil at stimulating hair follicle stem cells), Keratinocyte Growth Factor for follicle regeneration, and Copper Peptides for scalp tissue remodeling.

Scalp rollers — 0.5 mm for home use (creates microchannels, improves topical delivery, stimulates local circulation); 1.0 mm for in-clinic professional microneedling.

What About Skin?

We are developing a targeted skin product line using cellular senescence science—clearing zombie skin cells and restoring cellular energy to the skin. Details coming soon at HappyMD.co.

Chapter 12 — Hair Restoration: Waking Up the Follicle's Living Chip

Each hair follicle is a tiny, energy-hungry factory. In hair loss, that factory shifts into "slow" or "sleep" mode; growth phases shorten, rest phases lengthen, and strands miniaturize.

Our approach is three-layered:

Signal — Tell the follicle to wake up. JXL-069 is a topical spray that delivers a metabolic "wake-up" signal to hair follicles without hormones or finasteride-type pathways.

Fuel — Give that signal something to work with. Scalp MODS serum adds mitochondrial and scalp-health ingredients: NAD+, PQQ, copper peptide, niacinamide, methylene blue, and hyaluronic acid. It's applied especially after microneedling when the skin channels are open.

Access — Open the door to the follicle. Scalp rollers (0.5 mm at home, 1.0 mm in clinic) create microchannels and a localized repair response, improving delivery of topicals.

We package this into three options so you don't have to design your own protocol:

Hair Essentials — "Home start." JXL-069 spray + 0.5 mm roller. For early thinning or budget-friendly entry.

Hair Pro — "Full home protocol." JXL-069 + Scalp MODS serum + 0.5 mm roller. For more robust home treatment, adding fuel to the signal.

Hair Clinical — "Home + in-clinic precision work." Hair Pro kit plus four in-clinic microneedling sessions using the 1.0 mm roller. For more advanced loss or those wanting maximum intensity.

We always remind you: hair grows slowly. You're usually looking at 3–6 months for visible change and 9–12 months for full benefit, with photos and measurements to track progress.

During that time, we continue to tune hormones, mitochondria, nutrition, and stress. Because a thriving scalp almost always reflects a thriving system.

Chapter 13 — Longevity and Healthspan: Adding Life to Your Years

Living longer is only helpful if you can actually live in that time. Longevity without healthspan is just more calendar days in a body that can't do what you want.

Your Living Chip's long-term plan depends on:

- How much damage it's exposed to (toxins, ultra-processed food, chronic stress, poor sleep).
- How strong its repair systems are (mitochondria, autophagy, senolytics, antioxidant defenses).
- How often you send "build and repair" signals instead of "store and inflame" signals.

We use "longevity" tools to tilt those odds in your favor:

- Daily cellular maintenance (Activate365, Mito365, Restore365) to support energy and sleep.
- Targeted senolytic and mitochondrial support (Renew365, MitoBoost Ultra, NAD+ PQQ Boost) to help clear senescent cells and fuel repair.

To keep it simple, we organize this into two main bundles:

Longevity Core — "Optimize." Activate365 + Mito365 + Restore365. Daily cellular tune-up: better energy, mitochondrial support, and sleep.

Longevity Premium — "Maximize." Everything in Core plus MitoBoost Ultra + Renew365. Adds stress resilience and senolytic longevity support.

But longevity is never just a supplement stack. It is the sum of:

- Your daily movement and muscle mass
- Your sleep quality and circadian rhythm
- Your food patterns and alcohol use
- Your stress load and relationships
- Plus smart, targeted tools layered on top

We're not trying to "hack" immortality. We're trying to give your future self more years where you can walk, think, travel, play, and contribute the way you hope you will.

Chapter 14 — IV Days and Intensives: When to Use Drips and Deep Service

Most days, your Living Chip thrives on consistent oral support: the products you take every morning and evening, plus the lifestyle choices you make all day.

But sometimes you want—or need—a deeper intervention:

- You're coming off a period of extreme stress or illness.
- You're preparing for or recovering from high-intensity performance (athletic event, surgery, big work push).
- You feel "run down" despite doing the basics.
- You want a bigger NAD+ or methylene blue dose than is practical by mouth.

That's when we reach for IV therapy.

What IV Therapy Does

IV infusions deliver nutrients, antioxidants, and cellular fuels directly into your bloodstream, bypassing digestion and achieving higher tissue levels faster.

Think of it like this:

- Oral support is like watering a plant daily.
- IV therapy is like giving the plant a deep, root-soaking rain once in a while.

Both are useful. Neither replaces the other.

Our IV Menu

We keep it simple with six core drips and a few add-ons:

NAD+ Boost — High-dose IV NAD+ (250 mg). For deep mitochondrial support, post-illness recovery, brain fog, or fatigue.

Methylene Blue+ — IV methylene blue (1 mg/kg) plus B-complex. For cognitive sharpness, mitochondrial efficiency, and antioxidant support.

Vitality Drip — Vitamin C (10 g), B12, magnesium, zinc. The "classic wellness drip." General immune and energy support.

Performance Drip — NAD+ (100 mg) + methylene blue + B-complex. The combo for physical or mental performance demands.

Immune Shield — High-dose vitamin C (25 g) + glutathione. For acute immune support or detox phases.

Executive Focus — NAD+ (150 mg) + methylene blue + B12. Brain-targeted drip for mental clarity and focus under pressure.

Add-ons you can add to any drip:

- Glutathione push — Extra antioxidant support
- Extra vitamin C (10 g boost)
- Ozone therapy (nasal/auricular)

- IM B12 shot

When to Schedule IV Days

- Once a month during high-stress or intense training phases.
- Quarterly as part of a longevity or wellness routine.
- As needed when you're recovering from illness, travel, or burnout.
- Weekly only if part of an intensive program (like GLP-1 Tier 3 Transform).

All IVs are administered by our trained nursing staff under physician protocols. Each session takes 30–90 minutes depending on the drip. We'll help you decide what makes sense based on your goals, schedule, and budget.

Chapter 15 — Staying in Version 2.0: Follow-Up, Labs, and Adjustments

You don't "finish" health. You stay in conversation with your body and adjust as life changes.

Once we've started you on a plan—whether it's GLP-1, TRT, longevity bundles, or hair restoration—we schedule regular check-ins to make sure the system is working for you.

What Follow-Up Looks Like

Monthly visits (or as scheduled in your program):

- Weight, body composition, and vitals
- Symptom check: energy, sleep, mood, appetite, libido, focus
- Medication or product adjustments if needed
- "How do you actually feel?" conversation

Labs (timing depends on your program):

GLP-1 programs: Baseline, then every 8–12 weeks or as indicated. Metabolic panel, lipids, HbA1c, kidney function, liver enzymes. Sometimes thyroid, vitamin D, B12.

TRT programs: Baseline, 8 weeks, then quarterly. Testosterone (total and free), estradiol, SHBG, hematocrit, PSA. Lipids, liver function, metabolic panel.

Longevity / Wellness programs: Baseline, then 6–12 months. Comprehensive metabolic panel, lipids, inflammatory markers, hormone panel as appropriate.

We're not just chasing numbers. We're looking at the whole picture: how you feel, how your body is responding, and whether your Living Chip is thriving or struggling.

Red Flags — When to Call Us Between Visits

Most side effects are mild and manageable, but some need immediate attention.

GLP-1 red flags:

- Severe, persistent nausea or vomiting (can't keep fluids down)
- Severe abdominal pain (especially upper abdomen radiating to back)
- Yellowing of eyes or skin
- Suicidal thoughts or severe mood changes

TRT red flags:

- Chest pain or shortness of breath
- Severe headache or vision changes
- Painful, prolonged erection (priapism)
- Swelling in legs or sudden weight gain

Methylene blue note for patients on SSRIs/SNRIs:

- At the 10 mg oral dose in Best 365 products, no cases of serotonin syndrome have been reported in the published literature. All documented cases involved intravenous surgical doses 50 to 500 times higher. As with any medication, if you experience confusion, agitation, rapid heart rate, or high fever, call your doctor

Always call if something feels "really wrong" even if it's not on this list.

When We Adjust or Pause

Your plan is not locked in forever. We might adjust if:

- Side effects outweigh benefits
- Labs show an issue (kidney, liver, blood counts, hormones)
- You've reached your goal and want to step down
- Life circumstances change (pregnancy planning, surgery, new meds, financial shifts)

You are never "stuck." We work together to find what serves your current life, not a textbook protocol.

Chapter 16 — Quick FAQ: Common Questions and Honest Answers

Q: How long do I stay on these products or medications?

It depends on your goal and your body's response.

- GLP-1 medications: Often 1–2 years for weight loss, sometimes longer if there are metabolic or cardiovascular benefits. We step down gradually, not abruptly.
- TRT: Usually long-term if you're on testosterone cypionate. NHTO/enclomiphene can sometimes be cycled.
- Daily cellular support products (UCOS line): Many people stay on these indefinitely because they support foundational energy and repair.
- Hair products: Usually 9–12 months to assess benefit, then ongoing if working.

We reassess every few months and adjust based on your life, goals, and budget.

Q: Are these products FDA-approved?

Some are, some aren't.

- Semaglutide (GLP-1) and testosterone cypionate are FDA-approved prescription medications.
- Enclomiphene (NHTO) is compounded and used off-label for male hypogonadism.
- Supplements like NAD+, PQQ, methylene blue (USP grade), B12, etc. are not FDA-approved drugs; they're dietary supplements or research compounds.
- JXL-069 and Scalp MODS are labeled "research use."

We stay within legal and ethical boundaries and always disclose what you're getting.

Q: Can I take NAD+ if I'm on other medications?

Usually yes, but we check your full medication list. NAD+ precursors are generally well-tolerated. Regarding methylene blue: the serotonin syndrome warnings you may have seen online are based on intravenous surgical doses (0.74 to 8 mg/kg), not the 10 mg oral dose in our products. There are no published cases of serotonin syndrome at oral supplement doses, including in patients taking SSRIs or SNRIs. We still review your full medication list as a matter of good clinical practice.

Always tell us every medication, supplement, and over-the-counter product you take.

Q: Will I gain the weight back after stopping GLP-1?

It depends on what habits you built while you were on it. GLP-1 medications lower appetite and make behavior change easier. If you use that window to practice better defaults—protein-rich meals, regular movement, consistent sleep, stress management—you have a much better chance of maintaining.

If you go back to the exact same environment and habits you had before, the weight tends to return. That's why we build lifestyle support into every program, not just medication.

Q: Is methylene blue safe?

At the oral doses we use (10 mg, delivered as 2 x 5 mg), methylene blue is safe and well-studied for mitochondrial support. For IV therapy (1 mg/kg), we screen carefully and supervise in clinic.

Key cautions:

- Serotonin syndrome concerns: The warnings about methylene blue and SSRIs, SNRIs, or MAO inhibitors are based on intravenous doses used in surgery, not the 10 mg oral supplement dose. In the entire published medical literature, there is only one reported case involving oral methylene blue, and that patient was on multiple serotonergic medications at doses well above normal. At the Best 365 recommended dose, the risk is essentially theoretical. If you are on any serotonergic medications, let your prescriber know so they have the complete picture. Do not exceed the recommended dose.

- It will turn your urine blue-green temporarily (this is normal and harmless).
- Some people notice a blue tint on their tongue or lips for a few hours.
- Rarely, mild nausea or headache.

We review your medication list before starting any protocol, including products containing methylene blue. This is standard good practice, not a sign of danger.

Q: Can I do hair restoration if I'm also on GLP-1 or TRT?

Absolutely. In fact, optimizing hormones, metabolism, and mitochondria often helps hair too. We can stack:

- GLP-1 + Hair Protocol
- TRT + Hair Protocol
- Longevity Bundle + Hair Protocol

We just coordinate timing, check for any contraindications, and make sure you're not overwhelming yourself with too many new things at once.

Q: How do I know if it's working?

We track both objective and subjective measures.

Objective:

- Labs (metabolic markers, hormones, inflammatory markers)
- Body composition (weight, body fat %, muscle mass)
- Photos (for hair, skin, physique changes)
- Vital signs (blood pressure, resting heart rate)

Subjective:

- How you feel (energy, mood, sleep quality, focus, libido, appetite, stress resilience)
- How you function (can you do the activities you want? Are you recovering faster?)
- How you see yourself (confidence, clarity, sense of vitality)

If the numbers improve but you feel worse, we adjust. If you feel better but the numbers don't budge, we investigate why and decide together what matters most. Health is not a lab report. It's a lived experience.

Q: What if I can't afford the full program?

We work with you. Options include:

- Starting with the simplest product stack (e.g., GLP-1 Pack 2 instead of Pack 1).
- Focusing on lifestyle first and adding products later.

- Using monthly payments or prepay discounts (3, 6, or 12 months save 10–20%).
- Prioritizing what will have the biggest impact for your specific situation.

We never want cost to be the reason you don't get healthier. Let's talk openly about what's realistic, and we'll build a plan that fits.

Q: Can I stop anytime?

Yes. You are never locked in. Some medications (like GLP-1 or TRT) should be tapered or stopped gradually with medical guidance, but you're not contractually or medically forced to continue anything indefinitely.

If a product, medication, or program isn't working for you—financially, physically, or emotionally—we talk about it and adjust. Your autonomy matters as much as the science.

Closing Thought

You've now read the entire Owner's Living Chip Manual.

You know:

- Your body has a Living Chip that responds to every signal you send.
- Small, steady upgrades beat heroic, short-lived efforts.
- Sleep, movement, food, and stress are your foundation—always.
- Targeted tools (supplements, medications, IVs, topicals) can help your chip run better, faster, and longer when layered on top of real habits.
- You're not broken, lazy, or behind. You're just learning the user manual no one gave you at birth.

Now it's time to write Version 1.0 of your own plan, try it, learn from it, and update it as you go.

Your Living Chip is listening. What signal will you send today?

References

[1] Conze, D., Brenner, C., & Kruger, C. L. (2023). Dietary supplementation with NAD+-boosting compounds in humans: Current knowledge and future directions. Nutrients, 15(9), 1977. https://doi.org/10.3390/nu15091977

[2] Aman, Y., Qiu, Y., Tao, J., & Fang, E. F. (2022). The role of NAD+ in regenerative medicine. Plastic and Reconstructive Surgery, 149(4), 593e-608e. https://doi.org/10.1097/PRS.0000000000008808

[3] Nature Metabolism Editorial Team. (2026, January 14). The differential impact of three different NAD+ boosters on metabolic health. Nature Metabolism. https://www.nature.com/articles/s42255-025-01421-8

[4] NMN.com Science Team. (2026, March 3). Scientists unveil results from human trial directly comparing three NAD+ precursors. NMN.com. https://www.nmn.com/news/scientists-unveil-results-from-human-trial-directly-comparing-three-nad-precursors

[5] Yoshino, M., Yoshino, J., Kayser, B. D., et al. (2025). Nicotinamide riboside and nicotinamide mononucleotide facilitate NAD+ synthesis via enterohepatic circulation. Science Advances, 11(12), eadr1538. https://doi.org/10.1126/sciadv.adr1538

[6] Li, X., Zhang, Y., & Wang, Z. (2022). NAD+ and its possible role in gut microbiota. Frontiers in Nutrition, 9, 917922. https://doi.org/10.3389/fnut.2022.917922

[7] Advanced Metabolic Research Team. (2025, October 12). Disruption of gut microbiota-mediated de novo NAD+ synthesis affects metabolic health. Advanced Science. https://doi.org/10.1002/advs.202506497

[8] Vivere Research Team. (2026, January 15). What is the first pass effect? NAD+ & liver metabolism. Vivere Life. https://www.viverelife.co.uk/blog/first-pass-effect-explained

[9] Biotech Innovation Press Release. (2024, September 1). New study demonstrates that SL-NAD+ delivers NAD+ into cells. BioSpace. https://www.biospace.com/press-releases/new-study-demonstrates-that-sl-nad-delivers-nad-into-cells

[10] Goldman Laboratories. (2025, October 26). Liposomal vs sublingual NAD+: Which absorption method works best? Goldman Laboratories Blog. https://goldmanlaboratories.com/blogs/blog/liposomal-vs-sublingual-nad

[11] Weghuber, D., Barrett, T., Barrientos-Pérez, M., et al. (2022). Semaglutide improves cardiometabolic risk factors in adults with overweight or obesity: STEP 1 trial. Diabetes, Obesity and Metabolism, 25(2), 468-478. https://doi.org/10.1111/dom.14891

[12] Rubino, D. M., Greenway, F. L., Khalid, U., et al. (2024). Semaglutide: 4-year weight loss and cardiovascular benefits. European Association for the Study of Obesity. https://easo.org/semaglutide-4-year-weight-loss-and-cardiovascular-benefits/

[13] Lingvay, I., Sumithran, P., Cohen, R. V., & le Roux, C. W. (2024). Long-term weight loss effects of semaglutide in obesity without diabetes. Nature Medicine, 30, 1432–1440. https://doi.org/10.1038/s41591-024-02996-7

[14] Kosiborod, M. N., Abildstrøm, S. Z., Borlaug, B. A., et al. (2025). Semaglutide and cardiovascular outcomes by baseline cardiometabolic risk. The Lancet, 395(10314), 1821-1831. https://doi.org/10.1016/S0140-6736(25)01375-3

About the Authors

Steven Warren, MD, DPA, is a triple board-certified physician with over 45 years of clinical experience. He practices longevity and regenerative medicine in the Salt Lake City area at the Regenerative Wellness Center and serves as medical director of Best 365 Labs.

Darren Lopez, MBA, is CEO and Co-Founder of Best 365 Labs. With over 23 years in the nutraceutical industry, he has designed more than 50 health and wellness products including the MODS MAX absorption technology platform.

Acknowledgments

To our patients—you asked the questions this booklet answers. To our families—you put up with us while we answered them. And to Twiddle Max—the tireless assistant who helped turn 45 years of clinical experience into something you can read in one sitting.

Available at HappyMD.co

www.ingramcontent.com/pod-product-compliance
Lightning Source LLC
LaVergne TN
LVHW011051110826
845149LV00015B/3459
9781972800089